GETTING STARTED WITH HEARING AIDS FOR SENIORS

A guide for seniors to understanding, Navigating and living with hearing loss and Tinnitus and having auditory insights with hearing Aids.

Dr Leslie Pipes

UNDERSTANDING HEARING LOSS IN SENIORS

Millions of individuals worldwide suffer from hearing loss, a widespread condition that is particularly common in older persons. According to estimates, one in three persons between the ages of 65 and 74 and nearly half of all adults over the age of 75 have hearing loss. A person's quality of life can be greatly impacted by hearing loss, which can make it challenging to maintain independence, engage in social activities, and communicate.

Conductive and sensorineural hearing loss are the two primary categories.

An issue with sound waves reaching the inner ear is the cause of conductive hearing loss. Earwax accumulation or other blockages in the ear canal, as well as injuries to the eardrum or middle ear bones, may be the cause of this.

Damage to the inner ear's hair cells, nerves, or the connections that link the inner ear and brain can result in sensorineural hearing loss. In elderly adults, this is the most prevalent type of hearing loss.

The following are the most typical signs of hearing loss:

Having problems hearing high-pitched noises; asking people to repeat themselves; turning up the volume on the television or radio excessively loudly; having trouble understanding discussions, especially in busy situations;

experiencing ringing or buzzing in the ears (tinnitus)

Seniors' hearing loss has a number of causes, such as:

Ageing: The most prevalent cause of hearing loss in older persons is age-related hearing loss, or presbycusis. It is brought on by aging-related modifications to the inner ear.

Loud noise exposure: Loud noise from machinery, work, or music can harm inner ear hair cells, resulting in hearing loss. ***Medical conditions:** Certain medical conditions, including diabetes, hypertension, and Meniere's disease, can raise the risk of hearing loss.

Medications: A number of drugs, including aspirin and several antibiotics, have the potential to induce hearing loss as a side effect.

Heredity: Genetic factors can also contribute to hearing loss.

Although having hearing loss might be difficult, there are lots

of things you can do to manage
it and lead a fulfilling life.

THE IMPACT OF HEARING LOSS ON SENIORS

Hearing loss is a common and often overlooked condition that can have a significant impact on the lives of seniors. It can lead to social isolation, depression, and even an increased risk of dementia. Here's a closer look at the impact of hearing loss on seniors:

Communication Difficulties and Social Isolation

One of the most immediate impacts of hearing loss is

difficulty communicating. Seniors with hearing loss may struggle to follow conversations, especially in noisy environments. This can lead to misunderstandings, frustration, and a reluctance to socialize. As a result, seniors with hearing loss may withdraw from social activities and become increasingly isolated.

Depression and Anxiety

The social isolation and communication challenges associated with hearing loss can contribute to feelings of depression and anxiety in seniors. They may feel embarrassed about their hearing loss and avoid social situations. This can lead to a vicious cycle of isolation and depression.

Cognitive Decline and Dementia

Studies have shown that hearing loss is associated with an increased risk of cognitive decline and dementia. This may be due to the decreased social interaction and mental stimulation that can result from hearing loss. Additionally, hearing loss may put extra strain on the brain, as it has to work harder to process sounds.

Falls and Safety Concerns

Hearing loss can also increase the risk of falls and other safety hazards. Seniors with hearing loss may not be able to hear warning sounds, such as car horns or alarms. They may also have difficulty balancing if they cannot hear their footsteps.

Overall Impact on Quality of Life

Hearing loss can have a significant impact on the overall quality of life of seniors. It can make it difficult to participate in activities they enjoy, maintain relationships, and live independently.

What Can Be Done?

There are a number of things that can be done to help seniors with hearing loss, including:

Early diagnosis and treatment: Early diagnosis and treatment of hearing loss can help to minimize the negative impacts. Hearing aids and other assistive devices can help to improve hearing and communication.

Social and family support: Seniors with hearing loss need the support of their friends, family, and caregivers. It is important to be patient, understanding, and accommodating.

Cognitive stimulation: Seniors with hearing loss should engage in activities that stimulate their minds, such as reading, puzzles, and games.

This can help to offset some of the cognitive decline that may be associated with hearing loss.

Fall prevention: Seniors with hearing loss should take steps to prevent falls, such as using handrails, removing clutter from their homes, and getting regular eye exams.

Hearing loss is a serious condition that can have a profound impact on the lives of seniors. By understanding the risks and taking steps to manage hearing loss, we can help seniors to live happy, healthy, and independent lives.

TYPES OF HEARING AIDS

Behind-the-ear (BTE) Hearing Aids

Behind-the-ear (BTE) hearing aids are the most common type of hearing aid. They are worn behind the ear and have a tube that runs to a speaker or receiver in the ear canal. BTE hearing aids are available in a variety of sizes and styles, and they can be custom-made to fit your ear.

Benefits of BTE hearing aids:

- They are versatile and can be used for a wide range of hearing loss levels.

- They are durable and can withstand wear and tear.

- They are easy to use and maintain.

- They can be upgraded with new technology.

- They are often more affordable than other types of hearing aids.

Drawbacks of BTE hearing aids:

- They can be visible and may not be as discreet as other types of hearing aids.

- They can be uncomfortable to wear for some people.

- They can feedback, which is a whistling sound that can be annoying.

- They can be more susceptible to moisture and dust.

Overall, BTE hearing aids are a good option for many people with hearing loss. They are versatile, durable, and easy to use. However, they may not be the best choice for people who want a discreet hearing aid or who are concerned about feedback.

If you are considering a BTE hearing aid, it is important to consult with an audiologist to discuss your options and find the right hearing aid for you. An audiologist can help you choose the right size, style, and features for your individual needs. They can also provide you with training on how to use and care for your hearing aid.

In-the-ear (ITE) Hearing Aids

In-the-ear (ITE) hearing aids are custom-made hearing aids that fit snugly in the outer ear bowl. They are available in a variety of sizes and styles, including full-shell, half-shell, and canal. ITE hearing aids are a good option for people with mild to moderate hearing loss who want a discreet hearing aid.

Benefits of ITE hearing aids:

- They are discreet and are not visible when worn.

- They are comfortable to wear and provide a good fit.

- They are easy to use and maintain.

- They can be custom-made to match your ear canal.

Drawbacks of ITE hearing aids:

- They may not be as powerful as behind-the-ear (BTE) hearing aids.

- They may not be suitable for people with severe hearing loss.

- They may be more susceptible to moisture and earwax.

- They can be more difficult to adjust than BTE hearing aids.

Generally, ITE hearing aids are a good option for people with mild to moderate hearing loss who want a discreet hearing aid. They are comfortable to wear and provide a good fit. However, they may not be as powerful as BTE hearing aids and may not be suitable for people with severe hearing loss.**

If you are considering an ITE hearing aid, it is important to consult with an audiologist to discuss your options and find the right hearing aid for you. An audiologist can help you choose the right size, style, and features for your individual needs. They can also provide you with training on how to use and care for your hearing aid.

In-The-Canal (ITC) Hearing Aids

In-the-canal (ITC) hearing aids are small, custom-made hearing aids that fit snugly in the lower part of the ear canal. They are a good option for people with mild to moderate hearing loss who want a discreet hearing aid. ITC hearing aids are smaller and less visible than behind-the-ear (BTE) hearing aids, and they are also less prone to feedback.

Benefits of ITC hearing aids:

Discreet: ITC hearing aids are very small and fit snugly in the ear canal, making them a discreet option for those who want to avoid the visibility of hearing aids.

Comfortable: ITC hearing aids are custom-made to fit the individual's ear canal, ensuring a comfortable and snug fit.

Effective for mild to moderate hearing loss: ITC hearing aids are suitable for people with mild to moderate hearing loss, providing amplification and clarity to improve hearing.

Drawbacks of ITC hearing aids:

Less powerful than BTE hearing aids: ITC hearing aids

are smaller than BTE hearing aids, which may limit their power and amplification capabilities for severe hearing loss.

Requires careful handling: Due to their small size, ITC hearing aids may require more careful handling and maintenance to avoid damage or loss.

May not be suitable for all ear shapes: The custom-made nature of ITC hearing aids may not be suitable for all ear shapes, potentially causing discomfort or fit issues.

Generally, ITC hearing aids offer a discreet and comfortable solution for people with mild to moderate hearing loss. Their small size and snug fit make them less noticeable, while their custom design ensures a comfortable wearing experience.

If you are considering ITC hearing aids, it is important to consult with an audiologist to discuss your options and determine the suitability of this type of hearing aid for your individual needs. An audiologist can assess your hearing loss, evaluate your ear anatomy, and help you choose the right size, style, and features for your ITC hearing aids. They can also provide you with training on how to use and care for your hearing aids properly.

Completely -In-The-Canal (CIC) Hearing Aids

Completely-in-the-canal (CIC) hearing aids are the smallest and most discreet type of hearing aid. They fit entirely inside the ear canal, making them virtually invisible when worn. CIC hearing aids are a good option for people with mild to moderate hearing loss who want a hearing aid that is not visible.

Benefits of CIC hearing aids:

Discreet: CIC hearing aids are the most discreet type of hearing aid available, making them an ideal choice for those who want to avoid the visibility of hearing aids.

Comfortable: CIC hearing aids are custom-made to fit the individual's ear canal, ensuring a comfortable and snug fit.

Easy to use: CIC hearing aids are relatively easy to insert and remove from the ear canal.

Drawbacks of CIC hearing aids:

Less powerful than BTE hearing aids: CIC hearing aids are smaller than BTE hearing aids, which may limit their power and amplification capabilities for severe hearing loss.

May require more frequent cleaning: Due to their location in the ear canal, CIC hearing aids may require more frequent cleaning to prevent earwax buildup and potential malfunctions.

May not be suitable for all ear shapes: The custom-made nature of CIC hearing aids may not be suitable for all ear shapes, potentially causing discomfort or fit issues.

Overall, CIC hearing aids offer a highly discreet and comfortable solution for people with mild to moderate hearing loss. Their small size and in-ear placement make them virtually invisible, while their custom design ensures a comfortable wearing experience. However, it is important to consider the potential limitations in power and cleaning requirements for CIC hearing aids.

If you are considering CIC hearing aids, it is crucial to consult with an audiologist to discuss your options and determine the suitability of this type of hearing aid for your individual needs. An audiologist can assess your hearing loss, evaluate your ear anatomy, and help you choose the right size, style, and features for your CIC hearing aids. They can also provide you with training on how to use and care for your hearing aids properly.

CHOOSING THE RIGHT TYPE OF HEARING AID

Selecting the proper kind of hearing aid is a crucial choice that will have a big influence on your life. Finding the ideal hearing aid for you requires taking into account your unique requirements and preferences because there is a large selection of styles, functions, and technologies to choose from. Here is a guide to assist you in navigating the process of selection:

1. Begin by consulting an audiologist: Make an appointment with an audiologist to talk about your lifestyle and communication needs, as well as to have your hearing loss evaluated. To choose the best kind of hearing aid for you, they will assess your hearing levels, ear structure, and general health.

2. Take into account the extent of your hearing loss: The four categories of hearing loss severity—mild, moderate, severe, or profound—are used to classify hearing aids. Your audiologist will assist you in assessing the degree of your hearing loss and make recommendations for the best kinds of hearing aids for your individual requirements.

3. Select the appropriate style of hearing aid: Behind-the-ear (BTE), in-the-ear (ITE), completely in-the-canal (CIC), and receiver-in-canal (RIC) are the four primary types of hearing aids. Every style has pros and cons, taking into account things like visibility, comfort, and power needs.

4. Assess functionalities and technologies: Many features and technology are included in hearing aids to help with communication and hearing. These could feature

Bluetooth connectivity for streaming music from smartphones or other devices, telecoils for compatibility with assistive listening equipment, and directional microphones for improved speech understanding in noisy surroundings.

5. Give comfort and usability top priority: Long-term wearing comfort and ease of use and maintenance are essential features for hearing aids. To determine which design and size best fits your ear canal, try on a variety of options. When selecting your hearing aids, take into account your dexterity and comfort level with small parts.

6. Consider your tastes and lifestyle: Take into account your daily routine and the settings you visit. Features like water resistance or noise suppression could be crucial if you're an active person or spend a lot of time in noisy places. Select a style of hearing aid that is less noticeable, such as CIC or RIC, if discretion is an issue.

7. Talk about insurance and cost: The cost of hearing aids can vary greatly based on the design, features, and technology. Consult your audiologist about pricing choices and look into insurance coverage to ascertain your financial obligations.

8. Look for trial periods and modifications: Before making a final choice, you can test out various models and features with the majority of hearing aid dispensers during trial periods. Work closely with your audiologist throughout the trial time to fine-tune the programming and make necessary adjustments to guarantee optimal performance.

Recall that selecting the best hearing aid is a customized procedure that should be dictated by your unique requirements as well as the experience of your audiologist. You can select a hearing aid that enables you to re-establish a connection with the auditory world with careful thought and assistance.

SELECTING AND FITTING HEARING AIDS

Choosing a hearing aids provider

Selecting a provider for your hearing aids is an important choice that can have a big impact on how well you can hear and how satisfied you are with them overall. This thorough information will assist you in choosing the best provider for your needs:

1. Request suggestions: Ask your friends, family, medical professionals, and support groups for referrals of trustworthy local suppliers of hearing aids. Get opinions about their knowledge, treatment of patients, and general level of service.

2. Verify your professional qualifications: Check the provider's credentials professionally and make sure the appropriate bodies have granted them a license and certification. Seek out audiologists who hold the Academy of Dispensing Audiologists (ADA) or Hearing

Instrument Specialist (HIS) credentials.

3. Look up information online: Investigate possible providers using the materials available online. Compare their services and offerings, visit their websites, and read reviews. Take note of their credentials, areas of expertise, and patient satisfaction scores.

4. Arrange meetings with experts: Arrange meetings with several suppliers in order to compile data and contrast their methods. Inquire about the evaluation procedure, suggested hearing aids, programming techniques, and continued support services during the consultation.

5. Assess rapport and communication style: Evaluate the provider's bedside manner, communication style, and capacity to clearly and understandably explain complicated issues connected to hearing. Make sure you get along well with them and are at ease speaking with them.

6. Take into account accessibility and location: Take into account the accessibility and location of the provider. Make sure they provide tele-audiology or home visits if you have mobility issues. Select a service provider whose scheduling options are convenient and fit your schedule.

7. Get information regarding costs and insurance coverage: Talk about insurance coverage and price options up front. Inquire about financing alternatives, payment schedules, and any possible out-of-pocket costs. Recognize the billing policies and the insurance verification process of the provider.

8. Examine warranties and trial periods: Before making a purchase, find out if there are trial periods available to try out various features and kinds of hearing aids. Inquire about the warranty coverage for any related maintenance or repair services as well as hearing aids.

9. Get input from current patients: Whenever feasible,

get in touch with the provider's current clients to find out what they think of their overall experience, level of care, and level of skill.

10. Make a thoughtful choice: Select the provider that best fits your needs, tastes, and budget after giving it some thought. Put your chosen provider's experience, patient-centered care, and easy rapport first.

Hearing Aid Evaluation

A hearing aid evaluation is a comprehensive assessment that aims to determine your hearing loss, identify suitable hearing aid options, and ensure you receive the best possible care. Here's a detailed overview of the hearing aid evaluation process:

1. Initial Consultation and Hearing Test:

- Consultation: The process begins with an initial consultation with an audiologist. During this meeting, the audiologist will gather information about your hearing loss history, lifestyle, communication challenges, and expectations for hearing aids.

- Hearing Test: You will undergo a comprehensive hearing test to measure your hearing thresholds, identify areas of hearing loss, and determine the severity of your hearing impairment. This may include pure tone audiometry, speech audiometry, and other specialized tests.

2. Discussion of Findings and Hearing Aid Recommendations:

- Review of Results: The audiologist will review the results of your hearing test and discuss them with you in detail. They will explain the nature and extent of your hearing loss and how it affects your daily life.

- Hearing Aid Options: Based on your hearing test results, lifestyle, and preferences, the audiologist will present you with suitable hearing aid options. They will explain the features, benefits, and limitations of each type of hearing aid.

- Consideration of Budget and Insurance: The audiologist will discuss pricing options, insurance coverage, and any out-of-pocket expenses associated with hearing aids. They may also assist you in navigating insurance claims and paperwork.

3. Hearing Aid Fitting and Programming:

- Ear Impressions: If you are a candidate for hearing aids, the audiologist will take ear impressions to create custom earmolds or earpieces that fit snugly in your ear canals.

- Hearing Aid Programming: The audiologist will program your hearing aids based on your hearing loss profile, lifestyle, and communication needs. They will fine-tune the settings to optimize sound quality and improve your hearing ability.

4. Training and Ongoing Support:

- Hearing Aid Demonstration: The audiologist will demonstrate how to insert, remove, and operate your hearing aids. They will provide you with detailed instructions on how to use the various features and functions of your hearing aids.

- Communication Strategies: The audiologist will discuss communication strategies to enhance your listening skills and reduce the impact of hearing loss in various situations.

- Follow-up Appointments: The audiologist will schedule follow-up appointments to monitor your progress, make adjustments to your hearing aids as needed, and address any concerns or questions you may have.

Throughout the hearing aid evaluation process, your audiologist will work closely with you to ensure your hearing aids are properly fitted, programmed, and adjusted to provide optimal hearing performance and improve your overall quality of life.

Programming your hearing Aids

Programming your hearing aids is a crucial step in the process of optimising your hearing experience and ensuring they function effectively to address your specific hearing loss. It involves adjusting the settings and parameters of the hearing aid to align with your unique hearing needs and preferences.

Importance of Hearing Aid Programming:

Proper programming of hearing aids is essential for several reasons:

1. Enhances Sound Quality: Programming ensures the amplification and processing of sound are tailored to your individual hearing loss, providing a more natural and balanced listening experience.

2. Improves Speech Understanding: By adjusting the gain and frequency response, hearing aids can be programmed to enhance speech intelligibility, making it easier to understand conversations in various environments.

3. Reduces Feedback: Programming can minimize or eliminate feedback, a whistling or buzzing sound that occurs when amplified sound escapes the ear canal and re-enters the microphone.

4. Personalised Listening:

Programming allows for customization of hearing aid settings based on your individual preferences and listening needs, such as adjusting volume, noise reduction, and directional microphones.

Steps Involved in Hearing Aid Programming:

The hearing aid programming process typically involves the following steps:

1. Initial Assessment: The audiologist will review your hearing test results, medical history, and lifestyle factors to understand your hearing loss and communication challenges.

2. Hearing Aid Selection: Based on your assessment, the audiologist will recommend appropriate hearing aid styles and features that align with your needs.

3. Ear Canal Measurements: Ear impressions or ear canal measurements may be taken to create custom earmolds or earpieces for a snug and comfortable fit.

4. Programming Software: The audiologist will utilize specialized programming software to adjust the various settings of your hearing aids.

5. Sound Optimization: The audiologist will fine-tune the amplification, frequency response, and other parameters to optimize sound quality and enhance speech intelligibility.

6. Real-Ear Measurement:

In some cases, real-ear measurement techniques may be employed to verify the performance of the hearing aids in your actual ear canal.

7. Feedback Reduction: The audiologist will adjust the microphone settings and feedback cancellation algorithms to minimize or eliminate feedback.

8. **Personalization**: The audiologist will work with you to personalize the hearing aid settings based on your preferences, listening environments, and specific needs.

9. **Verification and Refinement**: The audiologist will verify the effectiveness of the programming through listening tests and real-world scenarios. Adjustments may be made as needed.

10. Training and Education: The audiologist will provide you with comprehensive training on how to use and maintain your hearing aids effectively.

Ongoing Monitoring and Adjustments:

Hearing aid programming is an ongoing process that may require adjustments over time as your hearing needs evolve or listening environments change. Regular follow-up appointments with your audiologist are essential to ensure optimal hearing performance and address any concerns or questions you may have.

Caring for your Hearing Aids

Proper care and maintenance of your hearing aids are essential to prolong their lifespan, ensure optimal performance, and prevent costly repairs. Here are some essential tips for caring for your hearing aids:

1. Daily Cleaning:

- Clean the exterior: Use a soft, damp cloth to wipe down the exterior of your hearing aids, removing any dirt, dust, or earwax buildup.

- Clean the ear molds or earpieces: Regularly remove and clean the earmolds or earpieces to prevent earwax accumulation. Use a wax removal tool or mild soap and water.

- Clean the microphone and battery compartment: Gently clean the microphone opening and battery compartment to ensure proper functioning.

2. Handling with Care:

- Handle with care: Avoid dropping or mishandling your hearing aids as this can damage delicate components.

- Store properly: When not in use, store your hearing aids in their carrying case to protect them from dust, moisture, and damage.

- Keep away from extreme temperatures: Avoid exposing your hearing aids to extreme heat or cold, as this can affect their performance.

3. Moisture Protection:

- Minimise moisture exposure: Keep your hearing aids away from water, sweat, and humidity. Remove them before showering, swimming, or engaging in activities that may expose them to moisture.

- Use a dehumidifier: Consider using a dehumidifying kit or storage case to remove moisture from your hearing aids when not in use.

4. Battery Care:

- Use the correct battery type: Use only the battery type recommended by your audiologist.

- Change batteries regularly: Change batteries promptly when they run low to maintain optimal performance.

- Store batteries properly: Store spare batteries in a cool, dry place away from extreme temperatures.

5. Regular Maintenance:

- Schedule regular checkups: Visit your audiologist for regular checkups and cleaning to ensure your hearing aids are functioning properly and adjusted as needed.

- Address issues promptly: If you notice any issues with your hearing aids, such as decreased sound quality or feedback, contact your audiologist immediately.

6. Follow Audiologist Instructions:

- Adhere to audiologist's recommendations: Carefully follow the instructions and recommendations provided by your audiologist regarding hearing aid care and maintenance.

By following these simple care and maintenance tips, you can extend the lifespan of your hearing aids, optimize their performance, and ensure a more enjoyable hearing experience.

LIVING WITH HEARING AIDS

Getting used to wearing hearing aids

Getting used to wearing hearing aids can take time and effort, but with patience and practice, you can overcome the initial challenges and enjoy the benefits of improved hearing. Here are some tips for getting used to your hearing aids:

1. Start slowly: Begin by wearing your hearing aids for short periods, gradually increasing the wearing time each day. This will allow your ears and brain to adjust to the new sounds and sensations.

2. Wear them in quiet environments: Initially, wear your hearing aids in quiet environments where there is less background noise. This will help you focus on the amplified sounds and get a better sense of how they work.

3. Practice with familiar sounds: Listen to familiar sounds, such as music, TV, or audiobooks, to help your brain adapt to the new auditory information.

4. Adjust settings with your audiologist: Work with your audiologist to adjust the settings of your hearing aids to optimize sound quality and address any specific concerns you may have.

5. Be patient and persistent: It takes time for your brain to relearn how to process sound and adapt to hearing aids. Don't get discouraged if you experience initial difficulties; be patient and keep practicing.

6. Seek support and advice: Discuss your experiences and concerns with your audiologist, friends, family, or support groups. They can provide valuable feedback and encouragement.

7. Use hearing aid accessories: Consider using hearing aid accessories, such as ear hooks, remote controls, or smartphone apps, to enhance your hearing experience and make adjustments easier.

8. Wear them consistently: Aim to wear your hearing aids consistently throughout the day, even in quiet environments. This will help your brain continue to adapt and improve your hearing over time.

9. Communicate with others: Let your friends, family, and colleagues know that you are getting used to wearing hearing aids. They can be more understanding and patient if they know what to expect.

10. Enjoy the benefits: As you get used to your hearing aids, you will start to notice the many benefits, such as improved speech understanding, reduced listening fatigue, and a greater sense of connection to your surroundings.

Remember, getting used to hearing aids is a journey, not a destination. Be patient, persistent, and work closely with your audiologist to optimize your hearing experience and enjoy the benefits of rediscovering the world of sound.

Communicating with others when you have hearing aids

Communicating with others can be challenging when you have hearing aids, but there are several strategies you can use to optimize your communication and make it easier to understand and be understood. Here are some tips for communicating effectively with hearing aids:

1. Position yourself strategically: When speaking with someone, position yourself face-to-face and slightly to the side of their speaking mouth. This will help you see their facial expressions and lip movements, which can provide additional cues to aid in understanding.

2. Ask for clarity: Don't hesitate to ask the speaker to repeat or rephrase something if you didn't understand it clearly. Most people are understanding and willing to accommodate your hearing loss.

3. Control background noise: Choose a quiet environment for conversations whenever possible. If you're in a noisy place, try to find a quieter spot or ask the speaker to move to a quieter location.

4. Use visual cues: In addition to listening, pay attention to the speaker's facial expressions, body language, and gestures. These visual cues can provide additional context and help you understand their meaning.

5. Take breaks: If you feel overwhelmed or fatigued during a conversation, take a short break to rest your ears and recharge. Let the speaker know you need a break and come back to the conversation when you're ready.

6. Use assistive devices: Consider using assistive listening devices, such as a headset or a telecoil, in public settings like theaters, conferences, or places of worship. These devices can amplify sound directly into your hearing aids, improving your ability to understand.

7. Educate others: Let your friends, family, and colleagues know about your hearing loss and how they can communicate effectively with you. Explain your specific challenges and preferences to help them understand how to best accommodate you.

8. Join support groups: Connect with other individuals who have hearing loss through support groups or online forums. Sharing experiences and strategies with others can provide valuable insights and support.

9. Be patient and assertive: Communicate your needs and preferences clearly and assertively to others. Don't hesitate to ask for adjustments or accommodations to ensure you can participate fully in conversations and activities.

10. Embrace technology: Utilize technology to enhance your communication, such as using video conferencing or real-time captioning apps, which can provide additional visual cues and support.

Remember, effective communication is a two-way street. By employing these strategies, you can empower yourself to communicate more effectively with others and enjoy more meaningful interactions.

Tips for seniors using hearing aids in different situations

Hearing aids can be a valuable tool for seniors, helping them to improve their hearing and communication in various situations. Here are some tips for seniors using hearing aids in different settings:

- **At Home:**

1. **Minimise Background Noise:** Turn down the TV, radio, or other sources of background noise when having conversations.

2. **Choose Quiet Environments:** Opt for quiet areas in your home for important conversations, such as a living room or bedroom.

3. **Face-to-Face Communication**: Position yourself face-to-face with the speaker to utilize visual cues and lip movements.

4. Ask for Clarification:
Don't hesitate to ask others to repeat or rephrase something if you didn't understand it clearly.

- **In Restaurants:**

1. Choose Quiet Locations: Request a table away from noisy areas like the kitchen or busy walkways.

2. Inform the Host: Let the host or server know you have hearing aids so they can speak clearly and at a moderate pace.

3. Face-to-Face Conversations: Engage in face-to-face conversations with your dining companions.

4. Minimise Background Noise: Ask the staff to turn down the music or TV if it's interfering with your ability to hear.

- **During Social Gatherings:**

1. Position Yourself Strategically: Sit near the speaker or in a quiet area where you can hear well.

2. Involve Multiple People:
Engage in smaller group
conversations rather than large
group discussions.

3. Take Breaks: If you feel
overwhelmed or fatigued, take
breaks from conversations to
rest your ears.

4. Use Assistive Devices:
Consider using assistive
listening devices, such as a
headset or a telecoil, to amplify
sound directly into your hearing
aids.

- **In Public Places:**

1. Choose Quiet Locations: When possible, opt for quieter areas in public places, such as libraries or parks.

2. Communicate with Confidence: Speak clearly at a moderate pace, facing the person you're addressing.

3. Ask for Assistance: Don't hesitate to ask for help from staff or volunteers if you need directions or assistance.

4. Utilise Technology: Use technology to enhance your communication, such as using video conferencing or real-time captioning apps.

ADDITIONAL TIPS:

1. Schedule Regular Check-ups: Visit your audiologist regularly for check-ups and adjustments to ensure your hearing aids are functioning optimally.

2. Carry Extra Batteries: Always have extra batteries on hand in case your hearing aids run low.

3. Clean and Maintain Your Hearing Aids: Follow the cleaning and maintenance instructions provided by your audiologist to keep your hearing aids in good condition.

4. Join Support Groups: Connect with other seniors who have hearing loss through support groups or online forums. Sharing experiences and strategies can provide valuable insights and support.

5. Be Patient and Persistent: Remember that getting used to wearing hearing aids takes time and effort. Be patient with yourself and keep practicing to improve your communication skills.

By following these tips and strategies, seniors can effectively use hearing aids in various situations, enhancing their communication and overall quality of life.

OTHER CONSIDERATIONS FOR SENIORS WITH HEARING LOSS

Assistive listening devices

Assistive listening devices (ALDs) can be a valuable complement to hearing aids for seniors with hearing loss, providing additional amplification and sound clarity in various situations. Here are some important considerations for seniors when choosing and using ALDs:

Types of ALDs:

1. Personal ALDs: These are handheld devices that amplify sound directly into the user's ears. They can be used in a variety of settings, such as theaters, conferences, and places of worship.

2. FM Systems: These systems use a transmitter and receiver to transmit sound wirelessly from a speaker or microphone to the user's hearing aids or a headset. They are particularly effective in noisy environments.

3. Infrared Systems: These systems use infrared light to transmit sound from a source to headphones or earphones. They are commonly used in theatres, museums, and other public places.

4. Audio Induction Loops: Also known as T-coils, these loops transmit sound through a magnetic field that is picked up by the T-coil in hearing aids or a neckloop. They are widely available in public places, such as theaters, airports, and libraries.

Choosing the Right ALD:

1. Consider your hearing loss: Consult with your audiologist to determine the type and severity of your hearing loss. They can recommend the most suitable ALDs for your specific needs.

2. Evaluate your lifestyle: Consider the environments and situations where you most need hearing assistance. This will help you choose the most appropriate ALDs for your lifestyle.

3. Test and compare: If possible, try out different ALDs to assess their sound quality, comfort, and ease of use.

4. Seek professional guidance: Work closely with your audiologist to select, program, and adjust ALDs to ensure they work effectively with your hearing aids.

Using ALDs Effectively:

1. Learn the operation: Familiarise yourself with the instructions and controls of your ALDs to use them effectively.

2. Position the receiver: Place the receiver or headset near your hearing aids or T-coil to ensure optimal sound reception.

3. Adjust settings: Adjust the volume and other settings to your comfort level and listening environment.

4. Seek assistance: Don't hesitate to ask for help from staff or volunteers if you have trouble using ALDs in public settings.

5. Combine with hearing aids: Use ALDs in conjunction with your hearing aids for maximum benefit, especially in challenging listening environments.

6. Regular maintenance: Maintain your ALDs according to the manufacturer's instructions to ensure their longevity and performance.

By carefully considering these factors and utilizing ALDs effectively, seniors with hearing loss can enhance their hearing experience and improve their communication in various settings.

HEARING LOSS AND TINNITUS

Hearing loss and tinnitus are two common conditions that often affect each other. Hearing loss is a partial or complete inability to hear sounds, while tinnitus is the perception of ringing, buzzing, or hissing sounds in the ears or head.

Prevalence of Hearing Loss and Tinnitus

Hearing loss is a prevalent condition, affecting approximately 5% of the population in the United States. Tinnitus is also common, with an estimated 15-20% of people experiencing it at some point in their lives.

Connection between Hearing Loss and Tinnitus

There is a strong link between hearing loss and tinnitus. In fact, about 90% of people with tinnitus also have hearing loss. The exact reason for this connection is not fully understood, but it is thought that damage to the hair cells in the inner ear, which are responsible for hearing, can also lead to tinnitus.

Symptoms of Hearing Loss and Tinnitus

The symptoms of hearing loss and tinnitus can vary depending on the severity of the condition. Hearing loss symptoms may include:

- Difficulty understanding speech, especially in noisy environments

- Needing to turn up the volume on the TV or radio

- Asking people to repeat themselves often

- Feeling like people are mumbling

Tinnitus symptoms may include:

- Hearing ringing, buzzing, or hissing sounds in the ears or head

- The sounds may come and go or be constant

- The sounds may be loud or quiet

- The sounds may be high-pitched or low-pitched

Treatments for Hearing Loss and Tinnitus

There is no cure for hearing loss or tinnitus, but there are treatments that can help manage the symptoms. For hearing loss, treatment options may include:

Hearing aids: Hearing aids can amplify sounds and make it easier to hear.

Cochlear implants: Cochlear implants are surgically implanted devices that can provide a sense of hearing to people with severe hearing loss.

For tinnitus, treatment options may include:

Sound therapy: Sound therapy involves using sound to mask or distract from the tinnitus sounds.

Cognitive-behavioral therapy (CBT): CBT can help people with tinnitus change their thinking patterns and reactions to the tinnitus sounds.

Medications: Certain medications may be used to help reduce the severity of tinnitus.

Living with Hearing Loss and Tinnitus

Living with hearing loss or tinnitus can be challenging, but there are ways to manage the symptoms and improve your quality of life. Here are some tips:

Get regular hearing tests: Regular hearing tests can help detect hearing loss early and allow for timely intervention.

Use hearing aids or other assistive devices: Hearing aids and other assistive devices can help you hear better and communicate more effectively.

Join a support group: There are many support groups available for people with hearing loss and tinnitus. These groups can provide you with information, support, and friendship.

Make lifestyle changes: Certain lifestyle changes, such as reducing stress and avoiding caffeine, may help reduce the severity of tinnitus.

If you are concerned about hearing loss or tinnitus, talk to your doctor or an audiologist. They can help you determine the cause of your symptoms and recommend the best treatment options for you.

HEARING LOSS AND MENTAL HEALTH

Hearing loss can have a significant impact on mental health, increasing the risk of various mental health conditions. Here's a comprehensive overview of the connection between hearing loss and mental health:

Impact of Hearing Loss on Mental Health:

Hearing loss can negatively affect mental well-being due to the social, communication, and emotional challenges it presents. Here are some of the ways hearing loss can impact mental health:

1. Social Isolation: Hearing loss can lead to social isolation and loneliness as individuals may avoid social interactions due to difficulty hearing or understanding conversations.

2. Communication Challenges: Communication barriers caused by hearing loss can lead to frustration, anxiety, and a sense of disconnection from others.

3. Reduced Self-Esteem: Hearing loss can negatively impact self-esteem and self-confidence, leading to feelings of inadequacy and social withdrawal.

4. Mental Health Conditions: Hearing loss is associated with an increased risk of developing mental health conditions such as depression, anxiety, and dementia.

5. Sleep Disturbances: Tinnitus, a common symptom of hearing loss, can interfere with sleep, leading to fatigue, irritability, and mood swings.

Factors Exacerbating the Impact:

Several factors can exacerbate the impact of hearing loss on mental health:

1. Severity of Hearing Loss: The more severe the hearing loss, the greater the potential impact on mental health.

2. Age of Onset: Hearing loss that occurs earlier in life can have a more significant impact on mental health development.

3. Individual Coping Mechanisms: Individuals with less effective coping mechanisms may be more susceptible to the negative effects of hearing loss.

4. Social Support: Lack of social support and understanding from family and friends can worsen the impact of hearing loss.

Strategies to Mitigate the Impact:

Fortunately, there are several strategies that can help mitigate the negative impact of hearing loss on mental health:

1. **Seeking Professional Help:** Consulting with an audiologist can provide diagnosis, hearing aid recommendations, and counseling.

2. **Using Assistive Technology:** Hearing aids, cochlear implants, and other assistive devices can improve

hearing and reduce communication barriers.

3. Joining Support Groups:
Connecting with others with hearing loss can provide emotional support and understanding.

4. Maintaining Social Connections:
Making an effort to maintain social interactions can combat isolation and improve mental well-being.

5. Engaging in Hobbies and Activities:
Participating in enjoyable activities can provide

a sense of purpose and reduce stress.

6. Seeking Mental Health Support: If experiencing mental health challenges, seeking professional counseling or therapy can be beneficial.

Hearing loss can have a profound impact on mental health, but with proper diagnosis, treatment, and support strategies, individuals can manage their hearing loss and improve their overall well-being. By addressing the social, communication, and emotional challenges associated with hearing loss, individuals can maintain a positive mental outlook and enjoy a fulfilling life.

Advocacy for seniors with hearing loss

Advocacy for seniors with hearing loss is crucial to ensuring they have access to the resources, services, and support they need to live fulfilling and independent lives. It involves raising awareness about hearing loss, promoting accessibility, and advocating for policies that address the needs of older adults with hearing impairments.

Importance of Advocacy:

Advocacy for seniors with hearing loss is essential for several reasons:

1. Raising Awareness: Hearing loss is often overlooked or stigmatized, making it crucial to raise public awareness about its prevalence, impact, and potential solutions.

2. Enhancing Accessibility: Advocates can work to make public spaces and services more accessible to individuals with hearing loss, including providing hearing loops, captioning services, and sign language interpretation.

3. Promoting Assistive Technology: Advocates can promote the use of assistive listening devices and hearing aids, ensuring seniors have access to the technology they need to hear effectively.

4. Influencing Policy: Advocacy can influence policy decisions at the local, state, and federal levels to support programs, funding, and research related to hearing loss in older adults.

5. Empowering Seniors: Advocacy can empower seniors with hearing loss to voice their concerns, advocate for their needs, and participate fully in society.

Strategies for Effective Advocacy:

Effective advocacy for seniors with hearing loss involves a multifaceted approach:

1. **Education and Awareness:** Educate the public, policy makers, and healthcare professionals about hearing loss, its impact, and available resources.

2. **Collaboration and Partnerships:** Collaborate with organizations serving seniors, hearing loss advocacy groups, and healthcare providers to amplify the voice of seniors with hearing loss.

3. Community Engagement: Engage with the community to raise awareness, organize events, and promote hearing loss screenings and prevention.

4. Policy Advocacy: Advocate for policies that support access to hearing healthcare, assistive technology, and affordable housing for seniors with hearing loss.

5. Support for Seniors: Provide direct support to seniors with hearing loss, including assistance with navigating resources, accessing services, and using assistive technology.

Examples of Advocacy Initiatives:

Here are some examples of advocacy initiatives for seniors with hearing loss:

1. Promoting Hearing Loss Screening Programs:

Advocate for the implementation of hearing loss screening programs in healthcare settings and community centers.

2. Supporting Hearing Aid Affordability: Advocate for policies that make hearing aids more affordable, such as insurance coverage and tax breaks.

3. Promoting Assistive Listening Devices: Encourage the installation of hearing loops and captioning services in public venues, such as theaters, libraries, and places of worship.

4. Supporting Hearing Loss Research: Advocate for increased funding for research on hearing loss prevention, treatment, and rehabilitation.

5. Ensuring Accessibility in Housing: Advocate for building codes and housing policies that make homes accessible to individuals with hearing loss.

6. Promoting Hearing Loss Awareness Events: Organize events and campaigns to raise awareness about hearing loss, its impact, and available resources.

7. Engaging with Policymakers: Attend town hall meetings, contact elected officials, and participate in public hearings to advocate for policies that support seniors with hearing loss.

8. Supporting Advocacy Organizations: Donate to and volunteer with organizations dedicated to advocating for hearing loss in seniors.

By implementing these strategies and engaging in advocacy initiatives, individuals, organizations, and communities can make a significant difference in the lives of seniors with hearing loss, ensuring they have the support and resources they need to thrive.

GLOSSARY OF HEARING TERMS

Here's a glossary of common hearing terms:

Audiogram: A graph that shows the results of a hearing test. It measures the softest sounds a person can hear at different pitches.

Auditory Neuropathy: A condition that affects the nerve pathways that connect the inner ear to the brain. It can cause problems with hearing and balance.

Assistive Listening Device (ALD): A device that helps people with hearing loss hear better. ALDs can be used in a variety of settings, such as theatres, conferences, and places of worship.

Cochlea: A snail-shaped structure in the inner ear that is responsible for hearing.

Conductive Hearing Loss: A type of hearing loss that occurs when sound is not able to travel properly through the middle ear. This can be caused by a variety of factors, such as earwax buildup, infection, or a tumour.

Decibel (dB): A unit of measurement used to express the intensity of sound.

Deaf: A person who has severe or profound hearing loss.

Earwax Removal Technician: A medical professional who specializes in removing earwax.

Eardrum: A thin membrane that separates the outer ear from the middle ear.

Eustachian Tube: A small tube that connects the middle ear to the back of the nose and throat. It helps to equalize the pressure in the middle ear.

Hard of Hearing: A person who has mild or moderate hearing loss.

Hearing Aid: An electronic device that amplifies sound and makes it easier to hear.

Hearing Dog: A trained dog that helps people with hearing loss by alerting them to sounds, such as door knocks and telephone rings.

Hearing Loop: A system that transmits sound directly to hearing aids or T-coils, which are tiny magnets that can be implanted in the inner ear.

Hearing Loss: A partial or complete inability to hear.

Inner Ear: The part of the ear that contains the cochlea and other structures responsible for hearing.

Interpreter-Sign language: A person who translates spoken language into sign language.

Irrigation: A procedure that uses water to remove earwax.

Low-intensity sounds produced by the inner ear: These sounds are known as otoacoustic emissions (OAEs) and can be measured with a sensitive microphone placed in the ear canal.

Outer Ear: The part of the ear that is visible on the outside of the head. It includes the pinna (the fleshy part of the ear), the auditory canal, and the eardrum.

Pinna: The fleshy part of the ear that is visible on the outside of the head. It is also known as the auricle.

Sensorineural Hearing Loss: A type of hearing loss that occurs when there is damage to the hair cells in the cochlea or to the nerves that carry sound from the cochlea to the brain.

Speech Audiometry: A hearing test that measures a

person's ability to understand speech.

Tinnitus: The perception of ringing, buzzing, or hissing sounds in the ears or head.

T-coil: A tiny magnet that can be implanted in the inner ear. It can be used to receive sound from hearing loops.

Tympanic Membrane: Another name for the eardrum.